Stress Busters

Easy to Use Outdoor Techniques

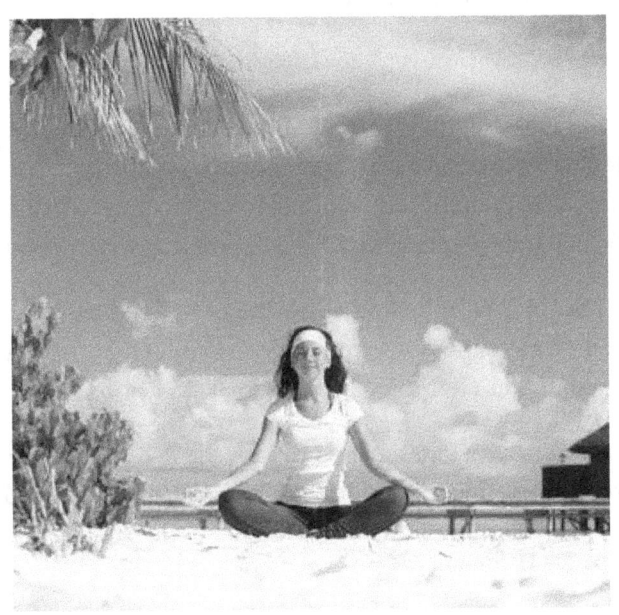

Healthy Learning Series

Dueep Jyot Singh

Mendon Cottage Books

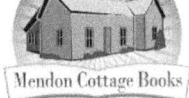

JD-Biz Publishing

Disclaimer

The information is this book is provided for informational purposes only. It is not intended to be used and medical advice or a substitute for proper medical treatment by a qualified health care provider. The information is believed to be accurate as presented based on research by the author.

The contents have not been evaluated by the U.S. Food and Drug Administration or any other Government or Health Organization and the contents in this book are not to be used to treat cure or prevent disease.

The author or publisher is not responsible for the use or safety of any diet, procedure or treatment mentioned in this book. The author or publisher is not responsible for errors or omissions that may exist.

Warning

The Book is for informational purposes only and before taking on any diet, treatment or medical procedure, it is recommended to consult with your primary health care provider.

Our books are available at

1. Amazon.com

2. Barnes and Noble

3. Itunes

4. Kobo

5. Smashwords

6. Google Play Books

Table of Contents

Introduction

Believe it or not, stress is definitely not a 21st-century phenomenon brought about by the rigors of struggling to survive in a harsh and unfriendly environment.

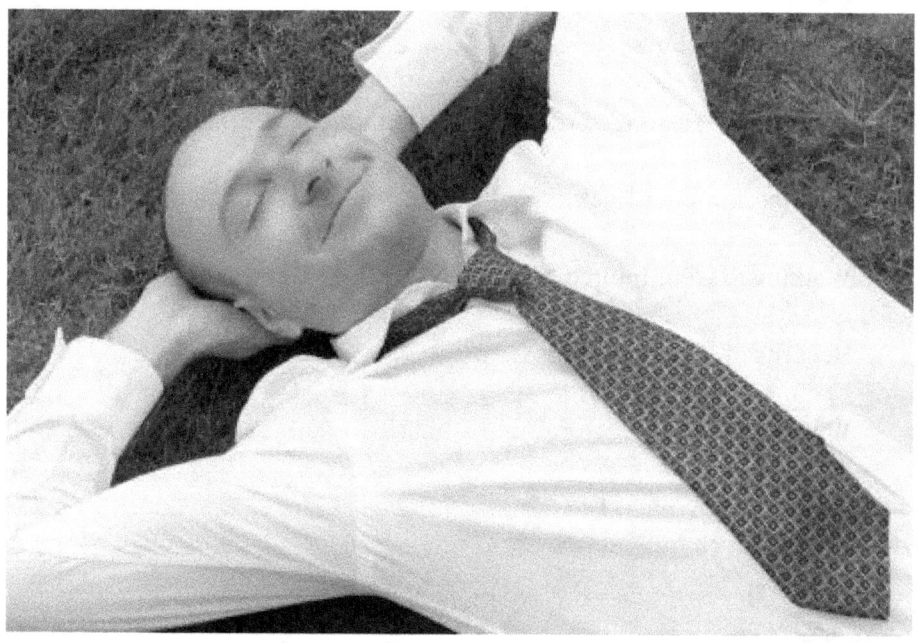

No stress, no tension, aaah, this is the life!

Stress has always been an important part and parcel of the human condition. That is why the old cliché was coined – All Work and No Play Makes Jack a Dull Boy. That was because man understood that fact that if he did not have any source with which he could relax and unwind, he would soon find himself gloomy, dull, lethargic and absolutely no interest in life, because for him, life would be bound to be full of just hard work and absolutely nothing else for which to look forward, at the end of the day.

And that is why he began to look at other options like singing, dancing, drama, painting, art forms in order to relax himself and forget about the stress, worry and tension in his life.

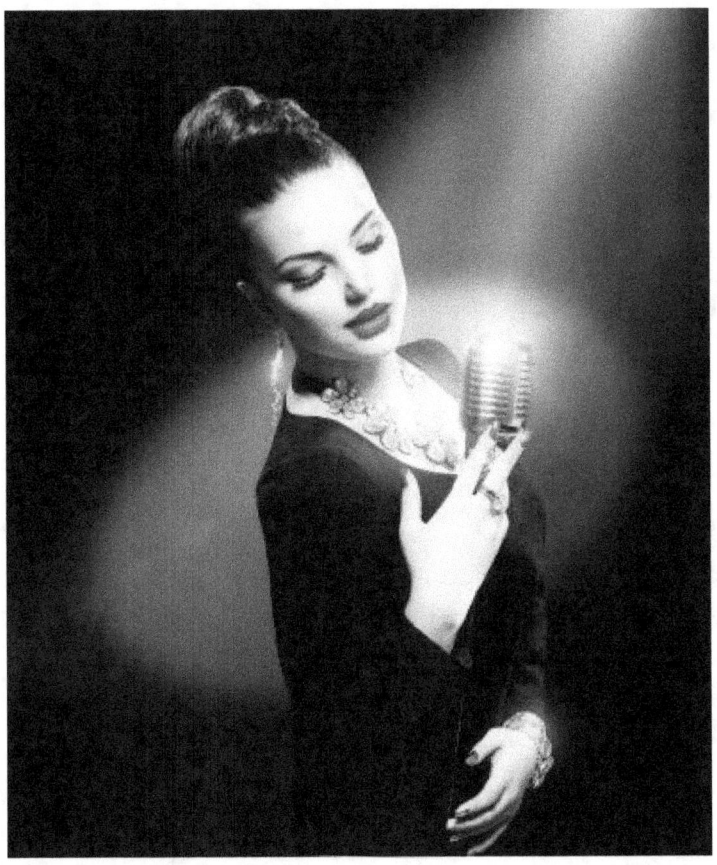

Singing is a relaxing activity, especially when you have to take in all that oxygen to hit the high notes!

This book is not going to tell you all about things you need to learn, because after all, who has the time to go to singing classes and dancing classes. Not I, because I am the busiest rat in the rat race. Neither may it be possible for you, because after all, you also have your own busy schedule and the fact that you are taking time out to read this shows that you have a little bit of breathing space before the next busy time in your day.

Laughter as an Exercise

Believe it or not, laughter is one of the most well-known and most effective of all the stress busters known to man. We have forgotten the power of laughter to keep us healthy. Just laugh out once, will you. You are going to notice that it is going to be either a restricted Ha ha or a socially polite giggle.

That is because the huge really enthusiastic and vigorous belly laugh is considered to be very noisy and not really accepted socially. I remember reading one of my favorite Georgette Heyer books – These Old Shades- where the hero, the dignified and aristocratic Duke of Avon closes his eyes daintily – talk about delicate sensibilities and sensitiveness in men –, when one of his friends bursts out in a natural and healthy guffaw of laughter.

Women, of course, would have considered loud laughter to be not at all dignified at all, and those rarified circles. They did not even speak above a whisper and their laughter or show of any amusement was constricted to just this polite and sickly simper.

So the sound of laughter began to disappear in the life of human beings, because it was supposed to be a loud noise in which only the supposedly lower classes indulged, especially when they were drunk.

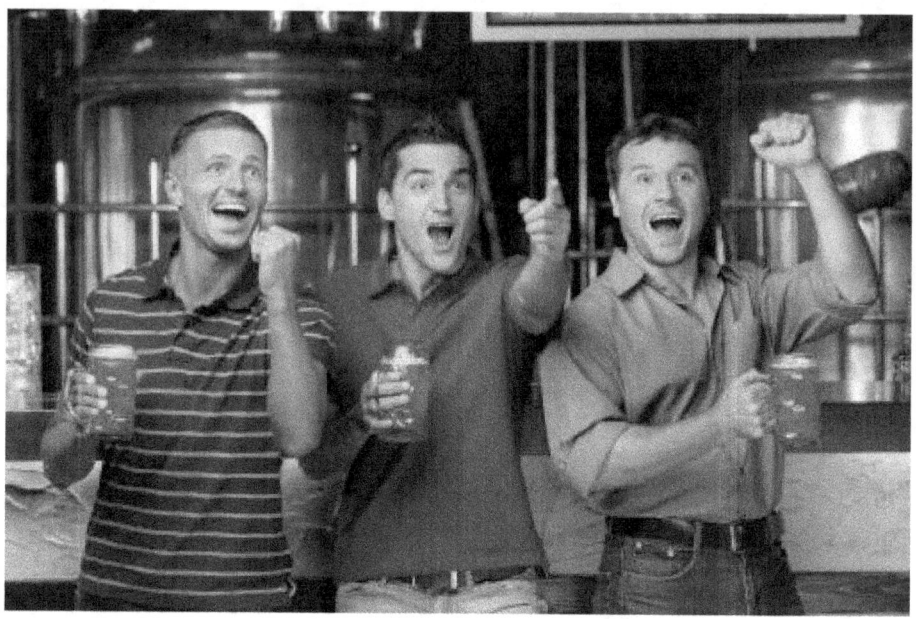

Luckily, the people of the 21st century have found out the benefits of laughter, especially when it is long and loud. It allows you to fill your lungs up with fresh oxygen. It lightens your heart, because what could be so amusing as a group of people with sober faces saying ha ha, in a laughter exercise in the park!

The first time this laughter club was made in our locality, a yoga trainer came there to teach people stress busting methods which including meditation and yogic exercises along with laughter therapy.

For us onlookers, who had not decided to join his classes, before we made up our minds that he was the goods, this was a good opportunity to see him in action. We did not bother much about the exercises and the meditation but we waited eagerly for his solemn "now we are going to start the laughter therapy. Close your eyes, take a deep breath, and laugh."

Everybody went ha ha ha ha in a doleful monotone, feeling half embarrassed. Naturally, the onlookers began grinning at that particular moment.

"My children, this is not the way to laugh," the guru spoke to his pupils, half of which were double his age. "You laugh deeply. You laugh loud. Now do it again, ha Ha."

A little louder yet still halfhearted ha ha ha ha, while the audience started giggling. Many of the pupils had this look of – I had better get out of here and quick, I think I am making a fool of myself, I have never laughed out loud, and here I have to laugh in public? Oh, help!"

"You laugh with all your heart," the guru would continue his instructions. "You have to laugh with deep breaths, taking in the magic of nature into your lungs, heart, body and soul. Put some spirit in your laughter, my children, ha ha. And loudly."

A little louder ha ha by a few who were still down but not out, but with no enthusiasm. The laughter in the audience is now audibly wholehearted, but the pupils are still trying their best to continue their laughter therapy.

This continued for a couple of days, with the audience getting visibly healthier and jollier thanks to the amount of pure oxygen being breathed in with our hearty bursts of laughter at our elders' possible embarrassment, discomfiture and chagrin , until one Elder protested.

"Guruji,"[1] he said pensively, "the only problem with the laughter therapy is that we have no reason to laugh out loud. If there was something to laugh at, we could laugh. We cannot laugh without any rhyme or reason without being considered to be totally mad!"

Naturally, this is the reasonable reason why so many people do not try out this method of stress busting outdoors. You could not even try this in your home because the neighbors would wonder what caused all that hysteria.

Nevertheless, laughter therapy, in the shape of natural, honest to goodness wholehearted loud laughter is an amazing stress buster. Try it out right now.

"But," you are going to say, "if I really want to laugh, I get my quota of laughter while watching a silly movie, or a sitcom."

Do you really think that laughter for about 30 seconds, done in a sitting position with your lungs cramped and in that closed atmosphere of your room is going to be any sort of therapy? Real beneficial laughter is always done outdoors, in a standing position. When your lungs get the opportunity to breathe in, and exhale the accumulated carbon dioxide in the outward ha ha, you may find yourself laughing long, loud, and naturally, and at nothing at all.

If you are still inhibited enough to feel shy, when you are doing this laughter therapy in a park with some companions, just look at their faces and look at the expressions of half sheepish embarrassment. If you do not burst out into

---

[1] Literally meaning Teacher Sir. The ji suffix is used extensively in the Indian subcontinent to show respect to somebody else than you or to someone you revere as a teacher or a mentor.

natural laughter at that particular moment, oh my friend, are you stressed out!

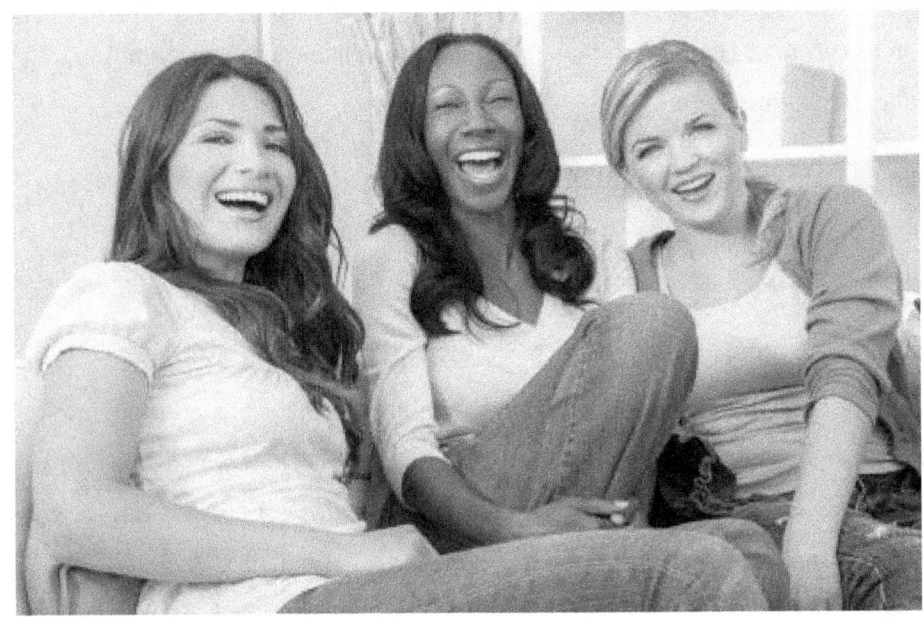

I remember one instance in the life and times of yours truly, when I asked the sibling about how he managed to cope with stress in his job, which often causes plenty of tension in him. As far as I know he has absolutely no other extracurricular interests like music, playing games, or even going outdoors for walks, with which he can relax.

This was his reply. He said that he learned this when he was just a beginner in his job, with other youngsters, -all of them bachelors, with no feminine influence or company for miles around – getting stressed out. They came back from work so tired that they had absolutely no other desire to do anything like play cards, gossip, and they were based in a place where there was no TV to which they could be glued and managed to pass the time.

So one day he just went out for a walk, in the area followed by the Mascot – affectionately named "Doggiedom"-when he found plenty of round stones on the ground. He did not have the time or the energy or the inclination to play fetch with the mutt.

So he just picked up two of the stones, and began clanging them together, making a really loud noise unto the mountains. And then he began to howl with his face raised up toward the sky.

The dog naturally appreciated all this noise, and joined in. When he stopped laughing, he found that he had found a really nice stress buster – laughter at some totally impulsive and half lunatic activity. His chief was so pleased at this new way of relaxation that he asked all the other officers to start their own Clanging Stone Club, with howls, noises and whistles.

Thirty three years have passed since then, but the clanging Stone club is a legend, to which every officer posted in that base has to contribute with weird noises, music, inarticulate songs, and sound effects, all accompanied by the clanging of stones to amuse his colleagues and superiors!

Believe it or not, this activity, though it sounds weird, is an extremely good stress buster, but you cannot do it in a crowded neighborhood. You may find the noise police coming in to haul you away in the nearest straitjacket. But that should not prevent you from the stress busting activity of laughter.

All you need to do is stand up, take deep breaths, and exhale, as if you are guffawing laughter. Make sure your neighbors know that you are doing laughter therapy, and are not suffering from a temporary fit of insanity.

Walking

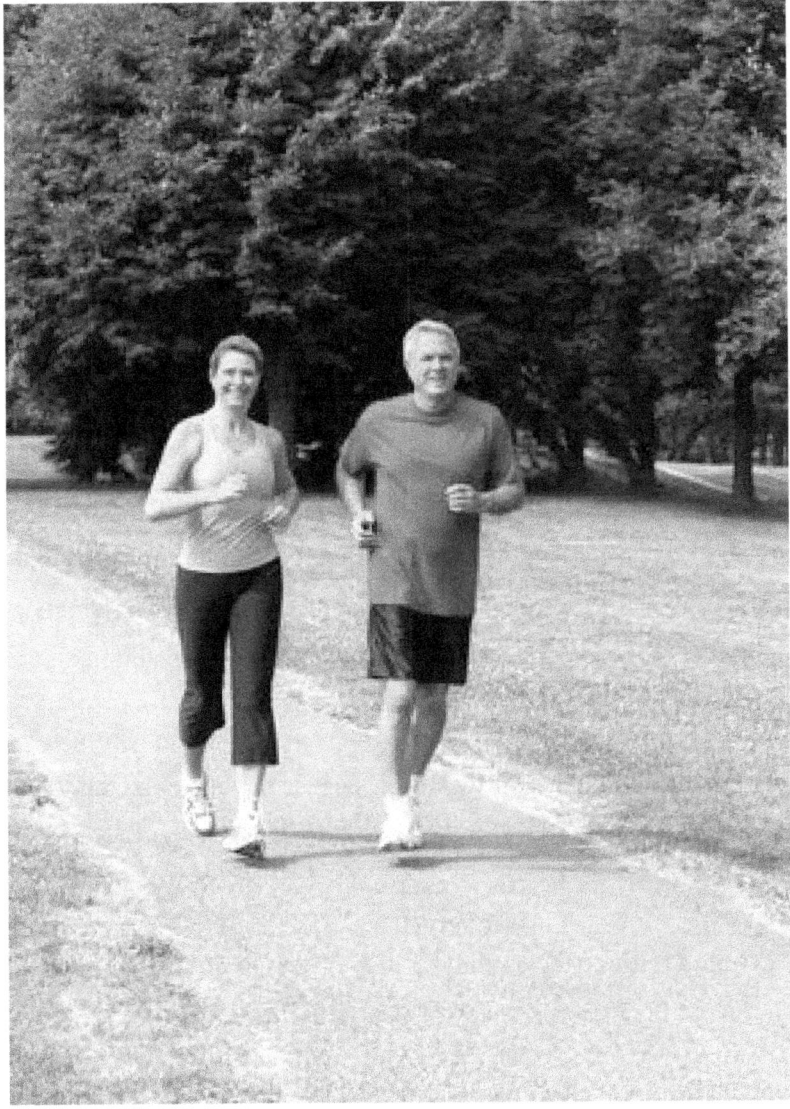

I was surprised to learn that one of my doctor friends considered walking to be one of the best stress busters. It was only in cases of emergency that he took his car to get to his hospital. Otherwise, he walked the three blocks from his house to his hospital, come rain come shine.

When I told him that he would get to his destination, his hospital room, exhausted, he said that the nurses had a standing order to keep a clean set of clothes ready for him, along with a glass full of cold and fresh lemon juice. This kept him going for the rest of the day, and even though he is in his 70s now, he has just one question for people who come to him with symptoms of aches, pains, and possible ill health.

"Do you do any walking?"

They do not. I do not, at the moment. And unless you are a fitness freak, it is possible that you also do not. Seriously speaking, just the thought of walking at a brisk pace, come rain come shine, but in the fresh air, makes me break out in a cold sweat, no pun intended. I just hate the clammy feeling of stickiness, especially when I am walking in the summer, even though it is relatively cool in the early mornings.

But here are the advantages of walking, because anybody can tell you that any good regimen of exercise, sincerely followed is going to be beneficial as it is going to work your heart and your lungs.

It is also going to force the cardiovascular system to deliver more blood and oxygen to feed the increased need of your muscles.

It makes the heart become more efficient, delivering blood and oxygen with each stroke.

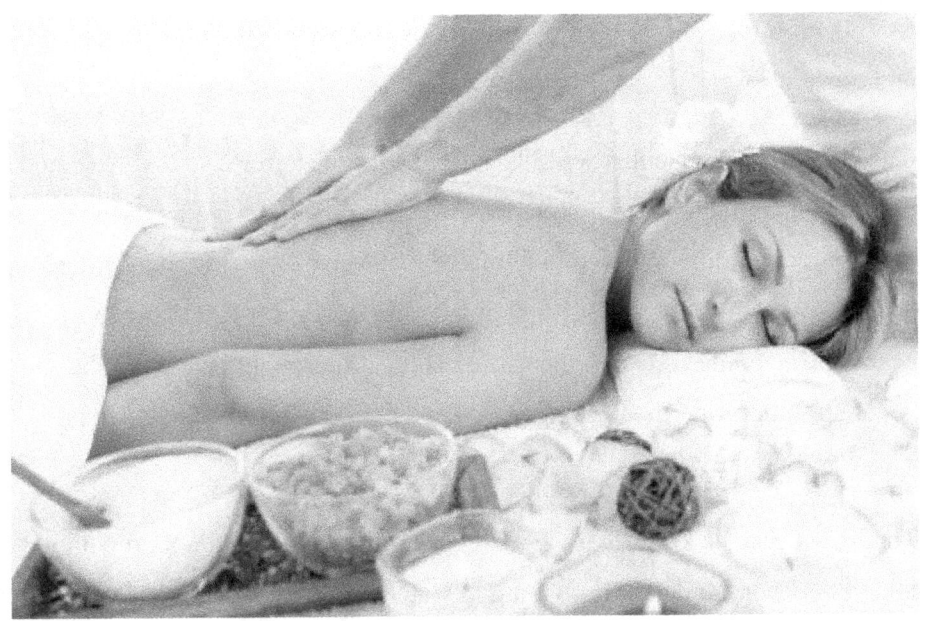

Massages can also get rid of stress and tension

There was a time when as a kid, I thought nothing of running, jumping, and walking through anywhere between five – 6 miles, every day in the green woods and mountains wherever father took his family on his peripatetic job.

And that is when I was the healthiest. I never suffered from any infectious sickness allowed in the body by a poor and weak immunity system and it was only when I grew up and had to come to the city, that I found myself suffering continuously from ill health.

It was an amusing fact that we children caught our measles, mumps and chickenpox when we had come down from the mountains into the plains during our annual holidays! That was when we did not have any opportunity to walk around, even though we spent our holidays in a wide-open garden and green city.

Our grandfather knew that we kids needed a lot of exercise so that we could be tired out enough not to be fractious when we needed to go to sleep. So early in the morning, he used to tell us to 23 Skidoo, scat, into the garden and outdoors, after breakfast, and not to come back until lunch. In the evenings, he made us water the garden and get thoroughly wet with the water sprinklers and the hosepipes. As Lin Yu Tang would say – Ah, Is This Not Happiness.

That is because he knew that we were forest imps and could not do without lots of Greenery and a daily soaking in water, having got used to that state of existence, in the mountains and tropical rainforests! We hated the city because according to us, this was a closed, concrete jungle where nobody could breathe anything fresh.[2]

Naturally, when we grew up our jobs became more and more sedentary, and we forgot about the walking we did when children and youths. This walking exercise made our heart more efficient, delivering pure blood and oxygen with every stroke.

But our sedentary lifestyle, piloting desks and hunched up in front of a table, was definitely not conducive to good health.

What we forgot is if the heart beats more slowly and more efficiently, the wear and tear on it, as well as on the arteries is going to be reduced. When

---

[2] Even today we associate greenery and lots of water with life and contentment, and dwindle away into nothingness, when we have to live in concrete jungles .

the heart pumps harder, the blood surges through the arteries. This discourages plaque, which is a substance that coats the arterial walls. This is the main cause of hindrance of blood flow and it also causes heart attacks.

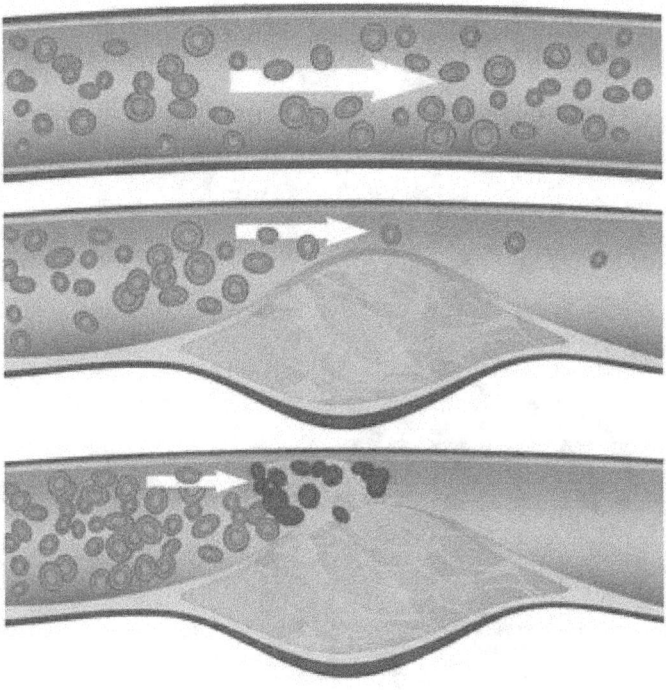

What we forgot is if the heart beats more slowly and more efficiently, the wear and tear on it, as well as on the arteries is going to be reduced. When the heart pumps harder, the blood surges through the arteries. This discourages plaque, which is a substance that coats the arterial walls. This is the main cause of hindrance of blood flow and it also causes heart attacks.

Also, any type of exercise is going to stimulate your brain to release endorphins. These are painkillers, with a similar structure to morphine.

The effect of these endorphins is like that of an analgesic. This is going to help control stress and tension.

That is the reason why so many people find an immediate improvement in their mood and a reduction of tension after a brisk physical workout, including walking.

One of the side benefits is that if you do a workout, you are going to be able to do more physical and mental work without tiring.

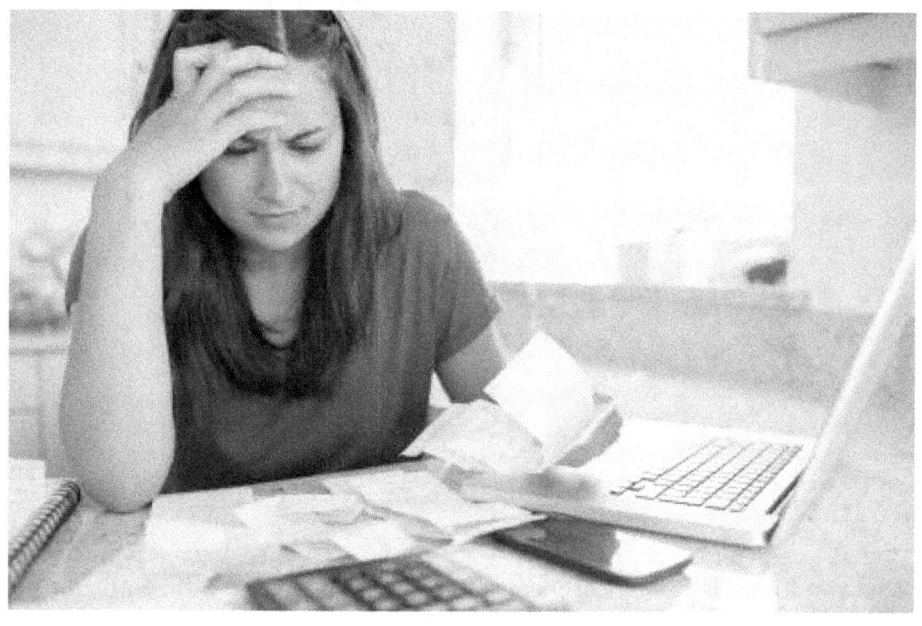

Mentally tired out, go for a walk.

Exercise also helps to build bones and improve the muscles. It strengthens them and makes your body more supple. A larger muscle is more efficient and flexible and is going to produce more energy.

Better muscles help us to work with less fatigue. More ever, stronger bones are going to ward off the dangers of osteoporosis when we hit our 60s and 70s.

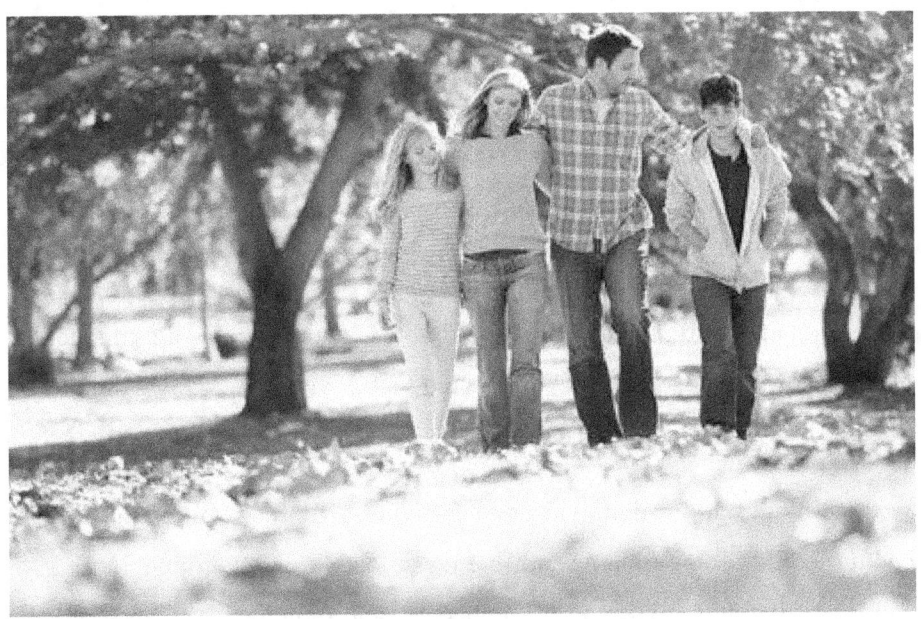

Make walking a family activity!

I remember my fitness freak uncle challenging me to walk like he did – 26 miles per day – but then he did not tell me that he had started out initially with walking just about 3 to 4 miles.

He told me to start slow, 3 miles per day in the park. Naturally this challenge was said in a tone of "I do not think you can do it, I just wanted to see if you could." Any of our respected elders taking that particular tone with us is quite capable of putting our backs up. And however they know our weaknesses and how to wind us up! They call it support and motivation.

Well, I started with 3 miles. When I finished that, around the park, I said, all right, I just need to show uncle dear what I could manage, and I did two more.

The next morning I woke up to stiff muscles. Getting to work was a pain, no pun intended. I had fallen into the pit of an enthusiastic exerciser. I had demanded too much of my flimsy and flabby muscles, which had not worked out for more than three decades!

No wonder people give up after just one exercise session. But that evening I was back in the park, mentally prepared not to let uncle have the satisfaction of saying "I told you so", and "I expected that of you, you really cannot do it!"

Within 15 days, my weight was down 3 pounds. My flabby thigh muscles had turned into something resembling legs. I was walking around 7 miles every evening with my zappin, switched on, and I jogging to a dance rhythm.[3].

That would have been good health heaven, but of course, that was the time when I had to get transferred out of that particular city to a place where there

---

[3] Try it out. Sumi Jo singing Arditi's Il Bacio
https://www.youtube.com/watch?v=24irhyFrQNI

were no gardens, no greenery, no place where you could be inspired to dance to the sound of *Sulle labbra se potessi dolce un bacio ti darei.*

And so I stopped walking, put on weight again and became a sedentary couch potato again.[4]

Remember that any sort of exercise is beneficial, but many of us definitely do not have the energy or the time to follow a regular regimen. Also, when we are alone, it is going to be difficult for us to sustain the motivation and willpower to keep on track.

That is why many of us decide to join gyms. But seriously speaking, not everyone can afford the cost of these expensive gyms and health centers. Sometimes they are also not very conveniently situated near your neighborhood or place of residence. A colleague of mine once told me that a gym was a very nice place where she could extend her professional network and social circles, but for me, gyms should be the places where you go to exercise instead of making business contacts!

Nevertheless, each to his own. And that is why I am advocating walking. That means you do not have to bother about any sort of gyms, all you need is a good pair of walking shoes. Walking can be done in your own garden or in a nearby park. As long as there is some wide open space, with plenty of greenery or like my cousin does, – she is a city mouse while I am a country mouse – she enjoys walking in her hustling bustling concrete jungle; walking can be done anywhere and at any time, but definitely not on a full stomach.

---

[4] Any excuse not to walk or exercise, especially when you are far away from under the Eagle eye of a vigilant uncle.

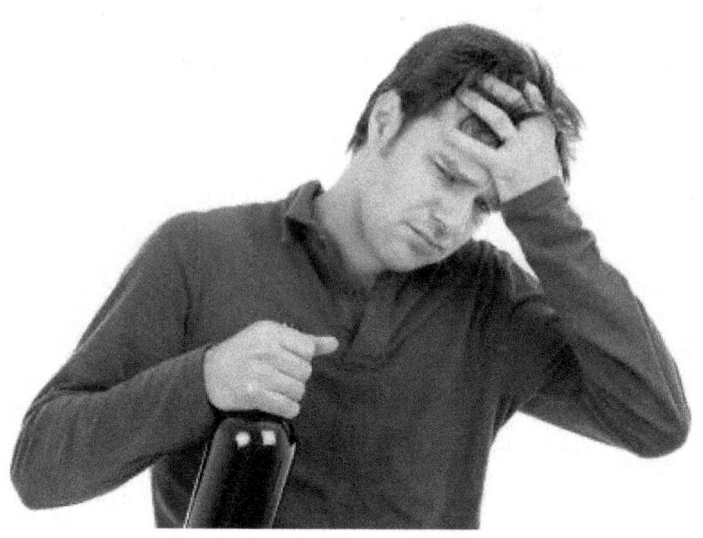

Alcoholic stimulants are definitely going to add to a state of stress and tension.

Exploring outside and adventuring

You can even walk on the pavements of your city, exploring the side roads. Forget about taking the nearest method of transport. Live life king size and do some adventuring. Who knows what secret adventure is waiting for you. Just round the corner, you may find a shop, which serves the most delicious food at really affordable and economical rates. You may find yourself finding amazing bargains, especially if you are a shopaholic.

That is why, as my cousin said, she does her walking with a money belt, with a little bit of money in it. That exercise routine also makes her indulge in her other love – hunting for bargains. Naturally, she never does her walking or shopping in areas which she does not know, at night.

When I first came to our city, which is called the city of Gardens, with a garden at every half mile, I was astonished to see a number of supposed walkers driving for about 8 miles in order to reach their favorite garden. They already had a group of all their friends waiting for them every evening. And this group was supposed to be walking and exercising.

I guess that was what they told their family members. Instead, they just sat there on the benches reciting memorized bits of verse and poetry, while we steady walkers walked briskly around them conscientiously happy that we were doing what we had come for, walking.

Well, I consider their version of "walking in the garden" to be an excellent way of stress busting.

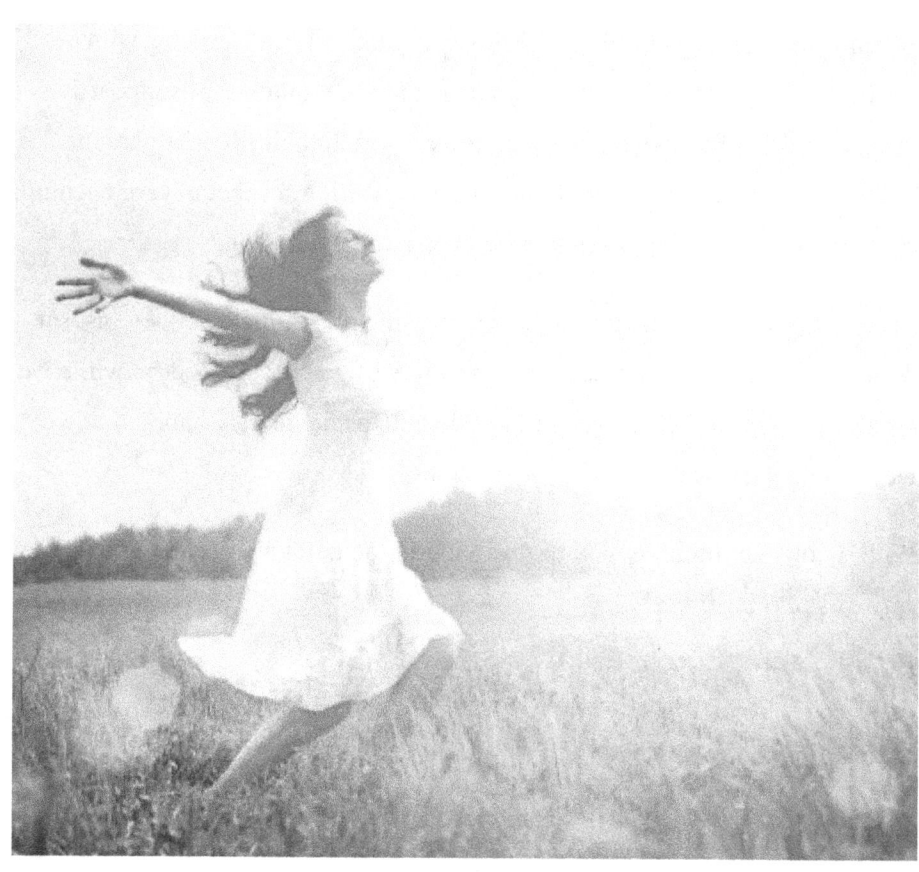

Proper Way to Walk

There is absolutely no ideal walking speed. What you feel is brisk at the moment may feel slow later, as your fitness increases. You have to start with a brisk but comfortable pace. What is more important is walking regularly and enjoying it and taking care of your proper posture, which is the basis of a healthy walking technique.

You have to walk tall with relaxed shoulders and focus on quicker steps let the stride length come naturally. Avoid looking down. Look forward without slouching or leaning forward at the waist.

The stomach muscles should gently be contracted to avoid an arched lower back. Some experts say an 85° bend at the elbow is good for a quick arm swing, which is going to mean quicker steps and a better walking speed.

It is best not to have a very short stride. To keep your steps long but comfortable push the foot back on the ground behind and extend the stride in back, not in front. Imagine placing your foot *in* the ground beneath you, not out in front. This is going to help in quicker steps and prevents over striding.

Cure for Loneliness

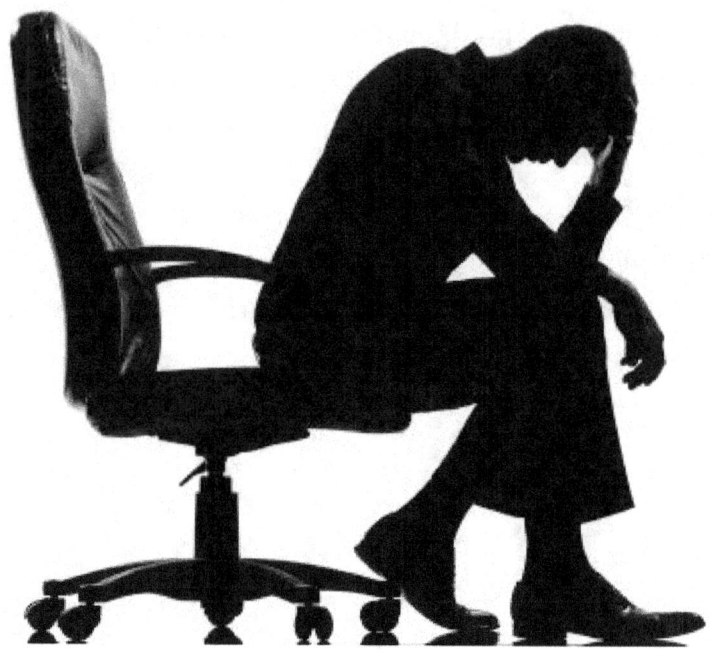

Stress, tension and depression may be factors contributing to loneliness and vice versa.

People who start walking regularly are soon going to find that it is addictive, and many of them cannot do without it. Those who walk regularly at a fixed time feel not only in communion with nature, but also build a silent rapport with others who were walking at the same time.

You may not talk to anyone but you are going to notice other people and feel at home and at one with society! That is the reason why walking is often considered to be a cure for loneliness and can be a boon to people living alone, especially elderly people. Parks are often a meeting ground for people of like interests – remember my "walking club" in the park, described above, where none of the members would ever see 60 again.

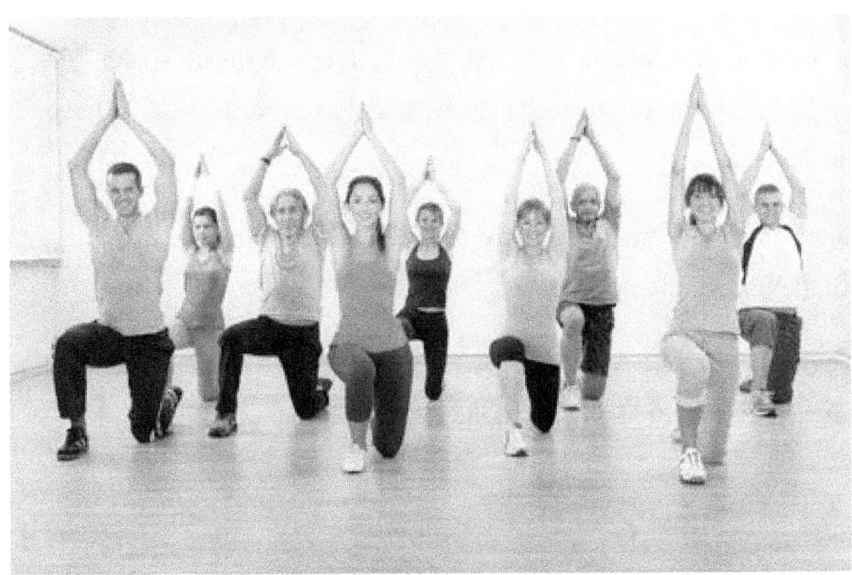

Joining any social group doing some sort of physical activity together is excellent in preventing stress.

Let me tell you something about why people, especially those in the older age group feel stressed. Their family members are often too busy and may not have enough of time to spend with them. Those unfortunate enough to have lost their spouses are going to be facing loneliness at home.

During their walking routine, they see other people. They may not talk to them but subconsciously they feel that they are a part of society and they have company. They may or may not make friends, depending on their personality, but they are soon going to feel much better and definitely not stressed.

The elders in my family start feeling uncomfortable when 5 o'clock strikes and there are people around them. It is time for their walk and here are all these people, preventing them from going out at five sharp. These people are so busy wasting time talking away about their lives and the great and glorious things they have done or they are about to do, or they could have done, as time fleets by.

The elders know the value of time. We do not. Because for us, we think we have all the time in the world.

This routine helps them feel that they have a say in their lives and schedules. Also, they want out after staying cooped up in the house and garden throughout the day!

Walking should be combined with a healthy diet and lots of water. Gentle warm-up exercises and easy stretches afterwards are going to keep you agile, supple, energetic and healthy. It is also going to stop you feeling any sort of stress because you are out in the sun, wind, and possibly rain!

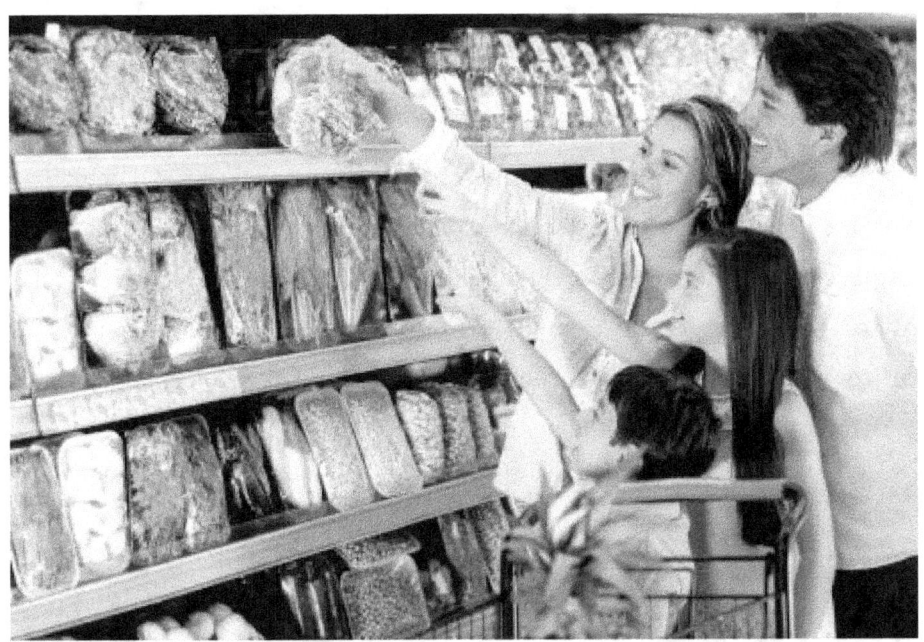

A healthy diet means a healthy family. Organic food is known to prevent stress, because it does not have artificial chemicals sprinkled on it. These chemicals are quite capable of changing your bio physiological makeup.

Walking for Healing

Also I found out by a physiotherapist friend, that walking is the best curative for people suffering from torn ligaments and muscular injuries. Of course they are not going to do their walking over long distances. But when I told her that this was told to me by my grandfather that the medical officers always recommended any injured warrior, – whether he was a soldier or an officer not to malinger on the bed, but go out and walk, this idea of healing is definitely not a modern idea or concept.

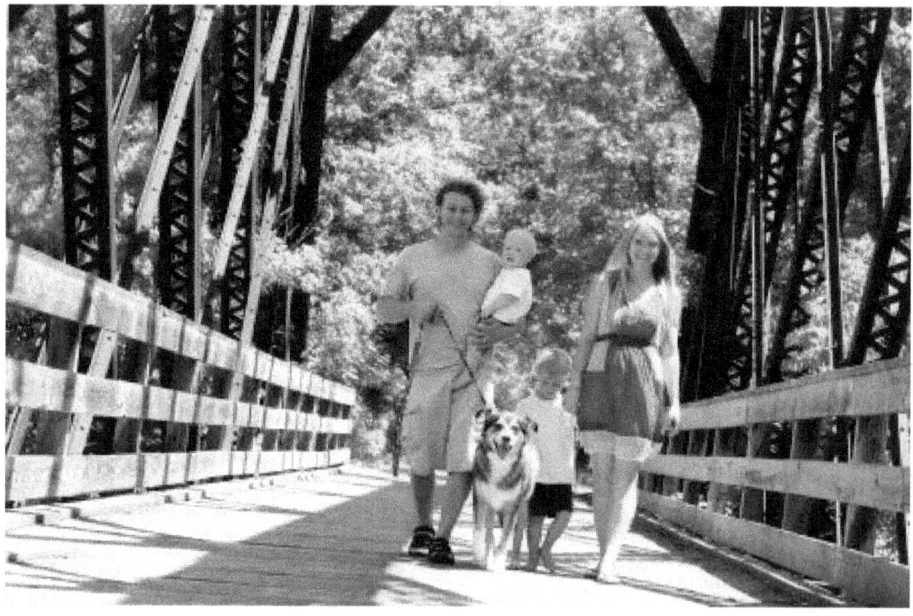

In Maurice Walsh's "The Spanish Lady, " the war weary and wounded hero who has been told to heal himself before he joins again for duty goes to the wide-open spaces where his uncle tells him to go out and walk and come back home, hungry.

Within a couple of months, the hero finds himself healthy, his ligaments and muscles strong and fit, and he in excellent spiritual, emotional mental and physical shape. This is what walking is going to do to you, mentally and physically. That is why I am talking about it as a stress busting medium.

Besides giving you all the benefits of exercise with the advantage of inhaling more fresh oxygen, walking is the most simple, inexpensive and easy to do stress busting technique available to man. Also, you are going to get all the good side effects of this exercise. Your body is going to be rejuvenated and your blood is going to be purified, with the removal of all the extra toxins.

Walking for Your Back

This walking is an aerobic exercise which is going to stimulate circulation and blood flow. Also, here is one point which many people do not know. It is literally possible to walk away from some types of back pain, no pun intended, just by walking.

This is because the injured ligaments, muscles, and discs are going to cure themselves. That is why more and more physiotherapist are advising walking as a therapy for lower back pain.

This is something which is literally true in my case. I began to suffer from lower back pain, because I kept sitting in front of the computer in a sedentary position without moving a muscle. And when I got up eight hours later, the muscles were stiff. No wonder my back was in very parlous shape.

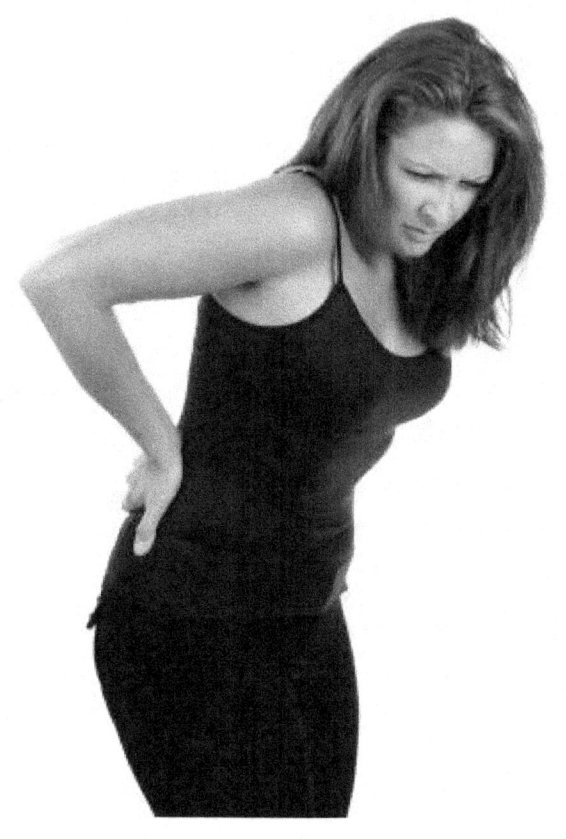

Did you know that lower back pain can be cured through walking?

But when I began to start walking, the muscles fell back into place. The oxygen supply began to cheer up and flow happily and enthusiastically through the muscles which had been cramped for eight hours at a stretch. And the back pain disappeared within five – six days of brisk walking. Try it out. And then you can say triumphantly, golly, my friend, you tell the truth, like it is! I promise not to say I told you so.

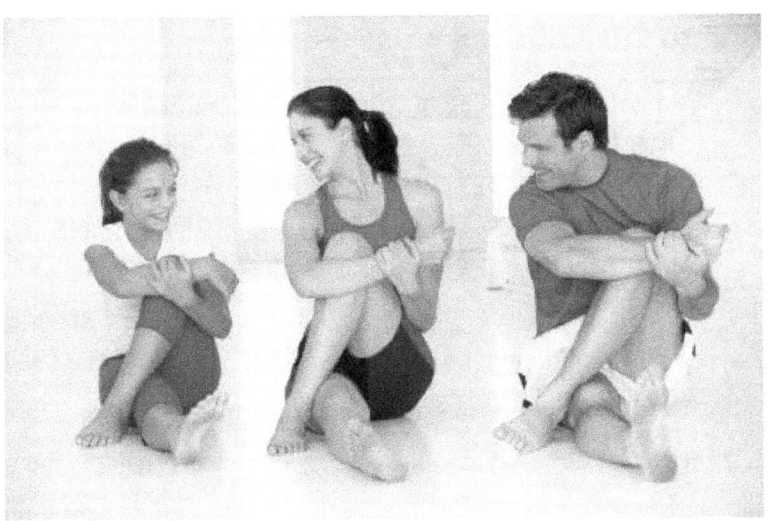

Light yoga exercises are also excellent to keep you mentally, physically, spiritually, and emotionally healthy!

Some back pain may be a symptom of a possible debilitating disease, but mostly back pain is not serious. This could be due to prolonged sitting in one position, bad posture, stress, lack of fitness, and also obesity. All these are definitely going to cured through walking, especially when you are getting these side benefits of this easy to do stress buster.

At first, you may need to go slow because a fast and brisk movement is going to create more upper trunk movement and an additional load on your back. A low load on your back is what makes swimming and walking just great exercises for sore backs.

Also, your walking is going to be done on level surfaces. Do not walk over rough ground. If possible, walk with a smooth and fluid motion. Do not jog, if you have back pain. Walk. That is because jogging is going to put more weight on your back than walking does.

Walking to Cure Injured Muscles

So how do you go about walking to cure injured muscles?

Now imagine your top priority is to build muscular endurance and to prevent loss of muscle mass, relieve pain and inflammation and increase the range of motion.

For this, you are going to do a little bit of walking on the first day, rest the second day. Do a little bit more of walking on the third day over a longer area. Rest the fourth day so that your muscles do not say, what is the matter with you, could not you give us a little bit of rest, after all, we are injured.

Remember that if you are suffering from sore muscles, you will need to continue walking, so that your muscles get used to this new exercise routine. That is why I say do not subject your body to any sort of enthusiastic trauma on the first day itself, so that your mind does not have an excuse not to exercise the next day.

For the best results, you are going to stretch after warming up a little bit. This is going to soothe and heal the sore muscles. Do some more stretching after you have finished your walk. We call it a full-fledged cat stretch.

That means you are going to stretch your arms above your head, or in any direct, and to the utmost of their limits. Open your mouth wide, and "yawn". You are getting all that accumulated carbon dioxide out of your system. And then slowly move your arms down, still stretching, and move your neck.

This is going to prevent any sort of muscular stress on your neck or on your shoulder muscles.[5]

A regular walking regimen is going to build up the endurance of your muscles in the leg, torso and pelvis, which support the spine. By warming up the muscles beforehand, walking can relieve the tightness and increase the mobility.

So if you have some chronic pain somewhere, the endorphins which are released during the walking session are going to help heal your body and mind and make you feel happier.

---

[5] The word for this particular action is called "Pandiculation"' "the act of stretching oneself". In yoga/Tantropathy, it is called angrai (uhng- rayee, which literally means yawning) . This is normally done, the moment you wake up and get out of your bed.

You can also make a pleasant , inarticulate and childish whhhheeee-ing sound or yawn while you are doing this stretching exercise because it is going to wake you up, thoroughly. The whole family enjoys doing this catlike stretching exercise along with early morning meeeheeeee -ings! And then we laugh because it sounds so silly.

By the way, this is definitely never done in public. I remember one of my junior trainees doing her stretching, yawning and wiggling at the end of a very tiring day, in the office, and the boss pulling her up with "what you think this is, a disco? This is not your papa's house." It was only later that she understood that angrais were not done in public because she was so used to doing them often, and without any self-consciousness whenever she wanted to stretch. Also, straightlaced old people considered this being done in front of males to be a straightforward invitation for conscious flirtation on the part of females. Men do not mind indulging in such a display anywhere when they are tired!

That is why chronic patients down the ages were always told to get out in the fresh air and stay there. Just by breathing in the fresh air, they would manage to get a fresher hold of life.

Benefits of Walking

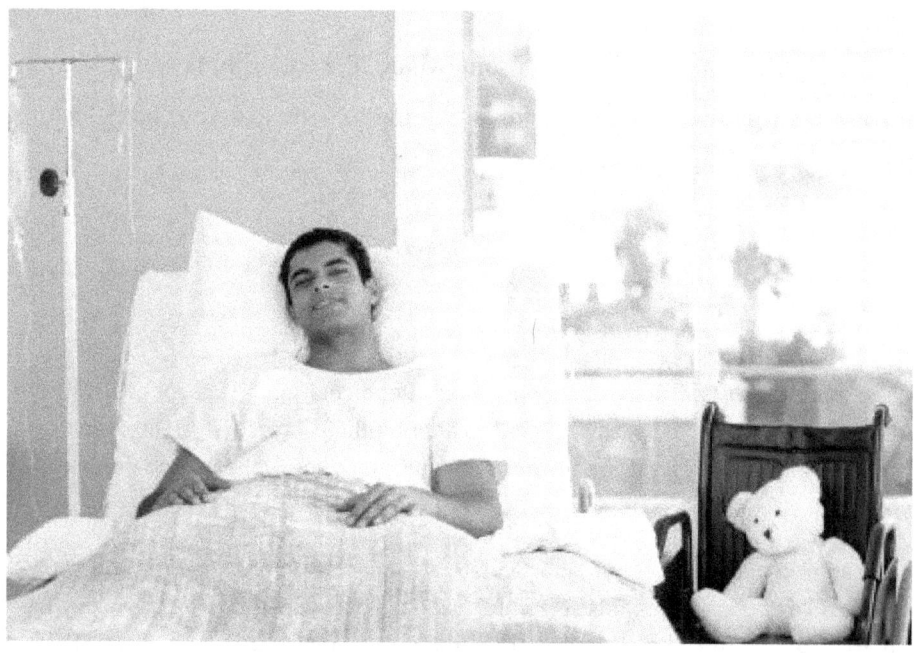

He will need to build up his stamina , again, when he comes out of the hospital with a good diet and walking.

Recent studies have shown that bedrest for more than one or two days is counterproductive as it is going to increase stiffness and weakness in your body and it is also going to create disability and depression, especially in patients.

Walking is also going to help in the state of your mind. When your body is fit, your blood pressure is low to normal. When the body is fit, it is going to be able to handle stress and strain better.

Dedicated walkers know that it is one of the best ways to sort out your problems. Walking makes the body feel good and helps the person deal more positively with his troubles and problems.

I normally do all my thinking over problems logistically and systematically while walking. I am not pacing around like a caged panther tearing holes in the carpet. I am doing my walking outside with the wind in my face. It is possible that consciously, I am not taking in my surroundings with all the noises and the distractions but subconsciously they are having a calming effect on my nerves.

When you are cooped up at home, personal problems are going to be magnified. But when you go out and see the people around you, and objectivity is going to come to your mind, and the problems fall into their proper perspective and their priority.

At times, at the end of the walk a person may realize that he was worried unnecessarily and tense for a matter which was basically very trivial.

When you are depressed or tense, you should try and go out for a walk rather than sit at home and brewed the walk is going to distract your mind and lighten your mood.

Now let me give you an example. I knew a friend who had this habit and tendency of blowing up every single problem into something unsurmountable and no wonder she was stressed out. Her main aim in life was saying "what am I going to do it this thing happens." There was a remote possibility of that thing happening ever in her life, but she loved to worry herself on the possibility that it could happen.

So there she was all stressed out worrying over what to do if she took out a mortgage, and she may not be able to pay back the money over a period of 30 years. This was a hypothetical question and not a top priority in her life at that time, but it was enough to stress her out.

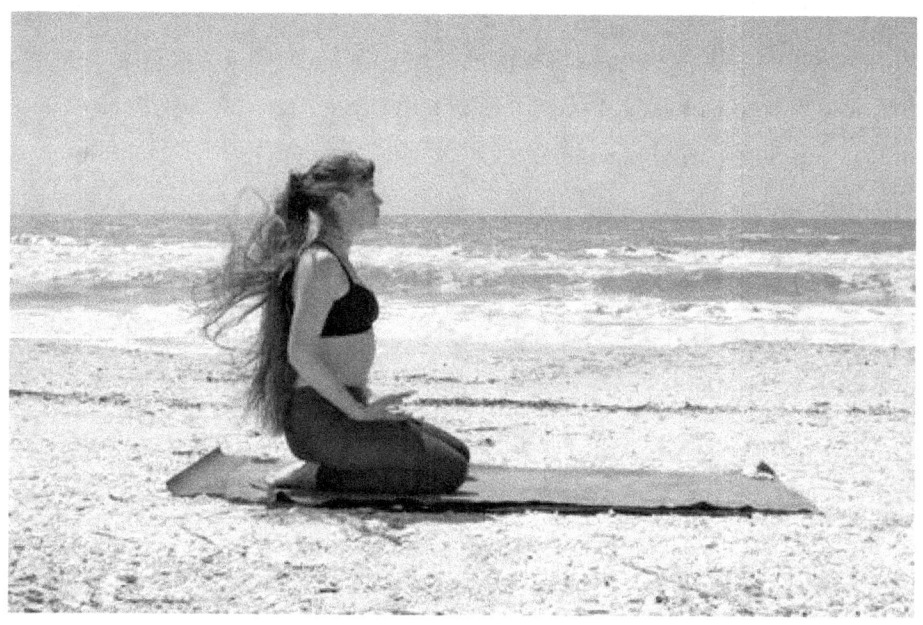

A day in the sun may also help prevent depression.

And then she went for a walk and she found a friend of her's who had gone completely bankrupt because she had not bothered much about her own financial wheeling and dealings. Suddenly it struck Emily that actually she was very fortunate when she compared herself with Sandra. Sandra had no financial resource open to her. Emily had a well paying job and money in the bank. She knew how to take care of her finances.

She also had a roof over her head while Sandra's stylish house had gone back to the bank to be auctioned in order to pay her debts, along with her car, expensive furniture and furnishings, jewelry, and paintings.

This immediately put things in proper perspective. In Emily's mind, things were clear now. With a little bit of management, she could manage to pay her mortgage. If she took out one, that could be done with proper and sensible planning. That was if she took out one, and she decided not to.

Now see how a little bit of calm and tranquil thinking helped her get rid of all that tension and unnecessary stress in her mind. Suddenly the gloom lifted from Emily' heart and when I saw her coming back, she asked me if I wanted to join her in a junk food binge?

I did, we ate lots of junk food and she has not thought about or talked about her mortgage, since then.

Ever since we found out that walking is the easiest way in which you can get rid of stress, and tension and put things in the proper perspective, whenever we feel we need to solve a problem, both of us head out for the wide-open spaces, in the midst of nature, chirping birds, buzzing insects, and greenery.

Walking is probably the best way in which you can raise high-density lipoprotein [HDL] and control serum cholesterol, which can be a risk for heart disease.

Walking and Acupressure

Many of us do not know that walking can also give the benefits of acupressure. Experts say that on the soles of the feet, there are certain points that are going to be pressed when you walk. These are instrumental in curing the body, as these are the controlling points of the liver, kidney, stomach, large intestines, small intestines, the bladder, the ureter and the suprarenal gland.

The Chinese knew all about these pressure points. Millenniums ago, they had special shoes built for walking, during which all these pressure points would be pressed gently. We do not know how people forgot about those shoes as time went by, and fashions changed, but any sensible person just needs to think about acupressure and walking related shoes.

For benefiting the most by walking, you have to be sure to get a really good pair of walking shoes, which should allow your feet to breathe. Do not wear tight shoes, because that means you are going to have sore feet and blisters at the end of the day.

It is better to walk on soft ground rather than on the road. Mornings and evenings are the best times when you should go out for a walk. That is because the weather is coolest, then especially in the summer season.

For maximum benefit, during walking, you can start gradually and increase the time slowly. An hour of walking is going to burn a lot of calories. But even lesser time is going to help you considerably. Instead of taking the car. You can walk to work or to the supermarket.

I remember a hilarious scene in the Classic Movie, "The Gods Must Be Crazy" where the director talks about how dependent we are on our vehicles while showing a lady coming out of her house, getting into her car, and driving to the letterbox just outside her driveway, which is just about 15 steps away from her door!

Walking for Weight Loss

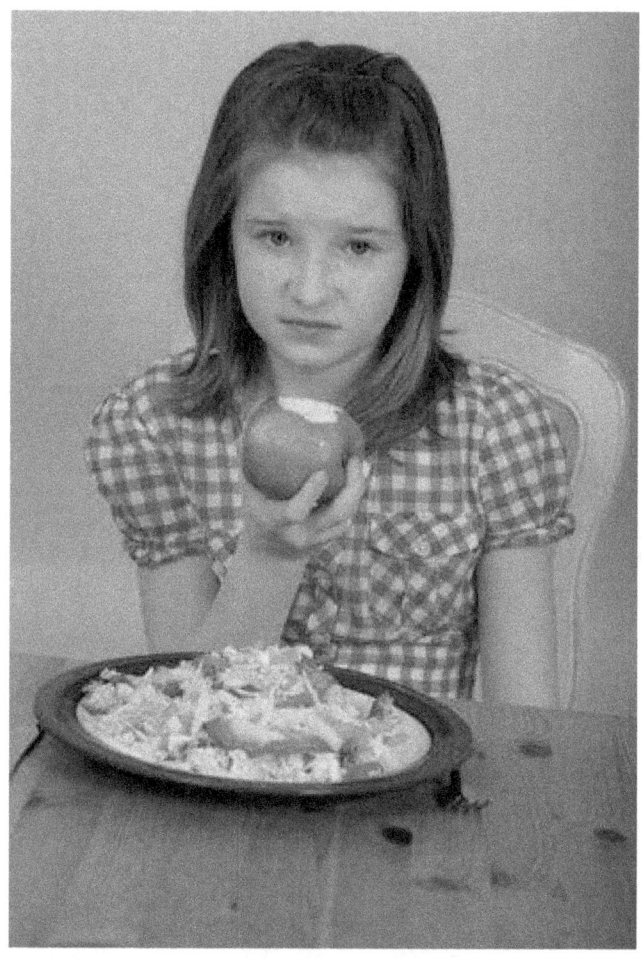

Do some walking to aide your dieting!

Walking combined with a careful diet is going to help you lose weight. As fitness improves, you are going to walk faster, and this is going to increase your calorie consumption.

More ever, walking increases metabolic rates and builds up your muscles. These are going to build to build up more muscles, and the more muscles you build, the more calories you are going to burn. So this is not a Catch-22 situation, but a beneficial circle.

German researchers have found out that under your feet exist certain points that make you lose weight automatically if you stimulate them. These points are going to force your body to get rid of the surplus fat. This can be done to an extent of losing 15 pounds in just six weeks, and that is without dieting or doing any extra exercises!

Conclusion

This book has given you plenty of information of natural and easy stress busters, including laughter therapy and walking. Not only is this going to keep you healthy, but you are definitely not going to be stressed out. If you follow the tips and techniques given in this book, you are going to feel healthier, happier, and even more social.

So try them out right now, Live Long and Prosper!

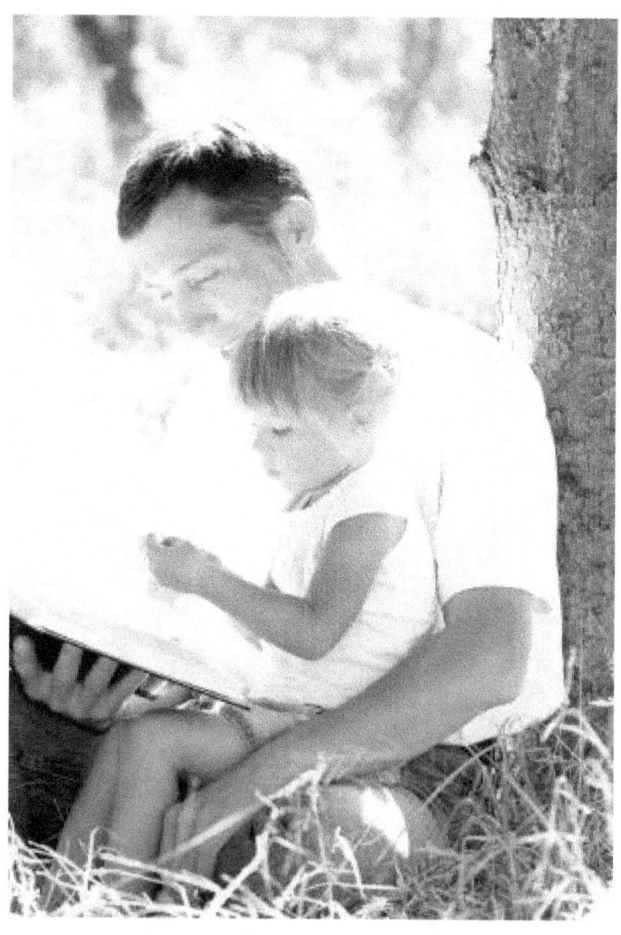

Author Bio

Dueep Jyot Singh is a Management and IT Professional who managed to gather Postgraduate qualifications in Management and English and Degrees in Science, French and Education while pursuing different enjoyable career options like being an hospital administrator, IT,SEO and HRD Database Manager/ trainer, movie , radio and TV scriptwriter, theatre artiste and public speaker, lecturer in French, Marketing and Advertising, ex-Editor of Hearts On Fire (now known as Solstice) Books Missouri USA, advice columnist and cartoonist, publisher and Aviation School trainer, ex-moderator on Medico.in, banker, student councilor ,travelogue writer … among other things!

One fine morning, she decided that she had enough of killing herself by Degrees and went back to her first love -- writing. It's more enjoyable! She already has 48 published academic and 14 fiction- in- different- genre books under her belt.

When she is not designing websites or making Graphic design illustrations for clients , she is browsing through old bookshops hunting for treasures, of which she has an enviable collection – including R.L. Stevenson, O.Henry, Dornford Yates, Maurice Walsh, De Maupassant, Victor Hugo, Sapper, C.N. Williamson, "Bartimeus" and the crown of her collection- Dickens "The Old Curiosity Shop," and "Martin Chuzzlewit" and so on… Just call her "Renaissance Woman") - collecting herbal remedies, acting like Universal Helping Hand/Agony Aunt, or escaping to her dear mountains for a bit of exploring, collecting herbs and plants and trekking.

Check out some of the other JD-Biz Publishing books

Gardening Series on Amazon

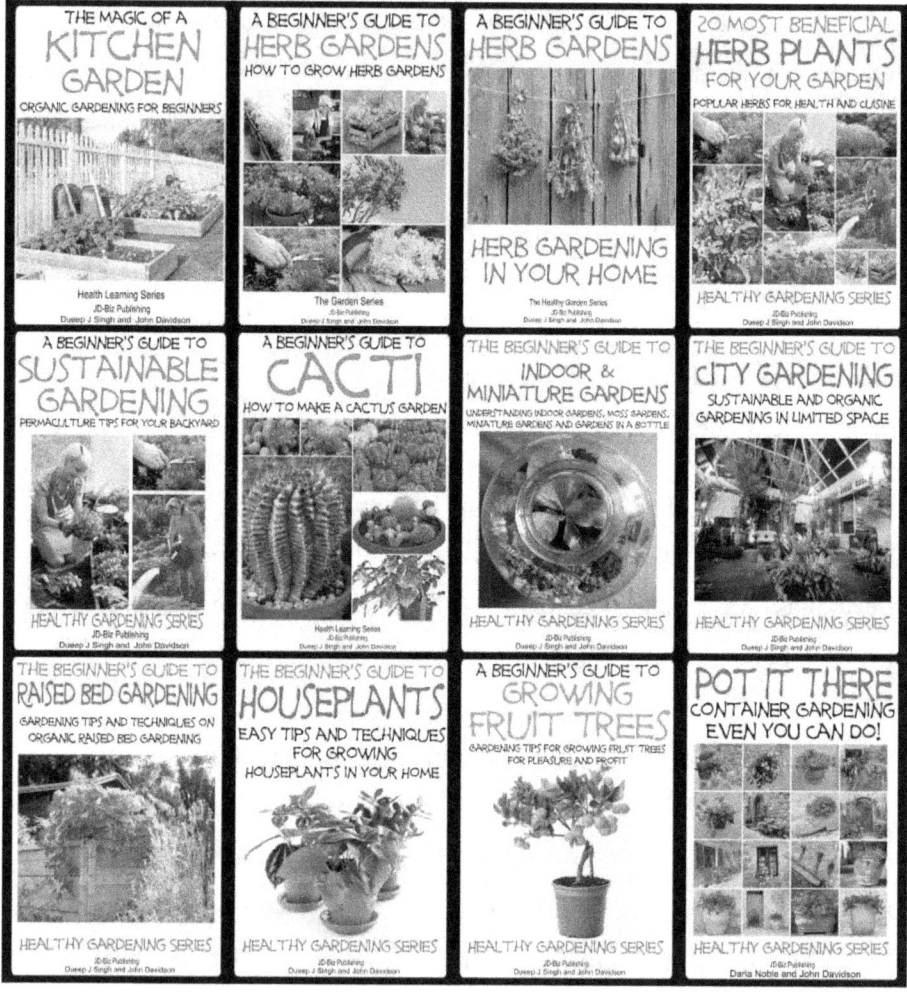

Health Learning Series

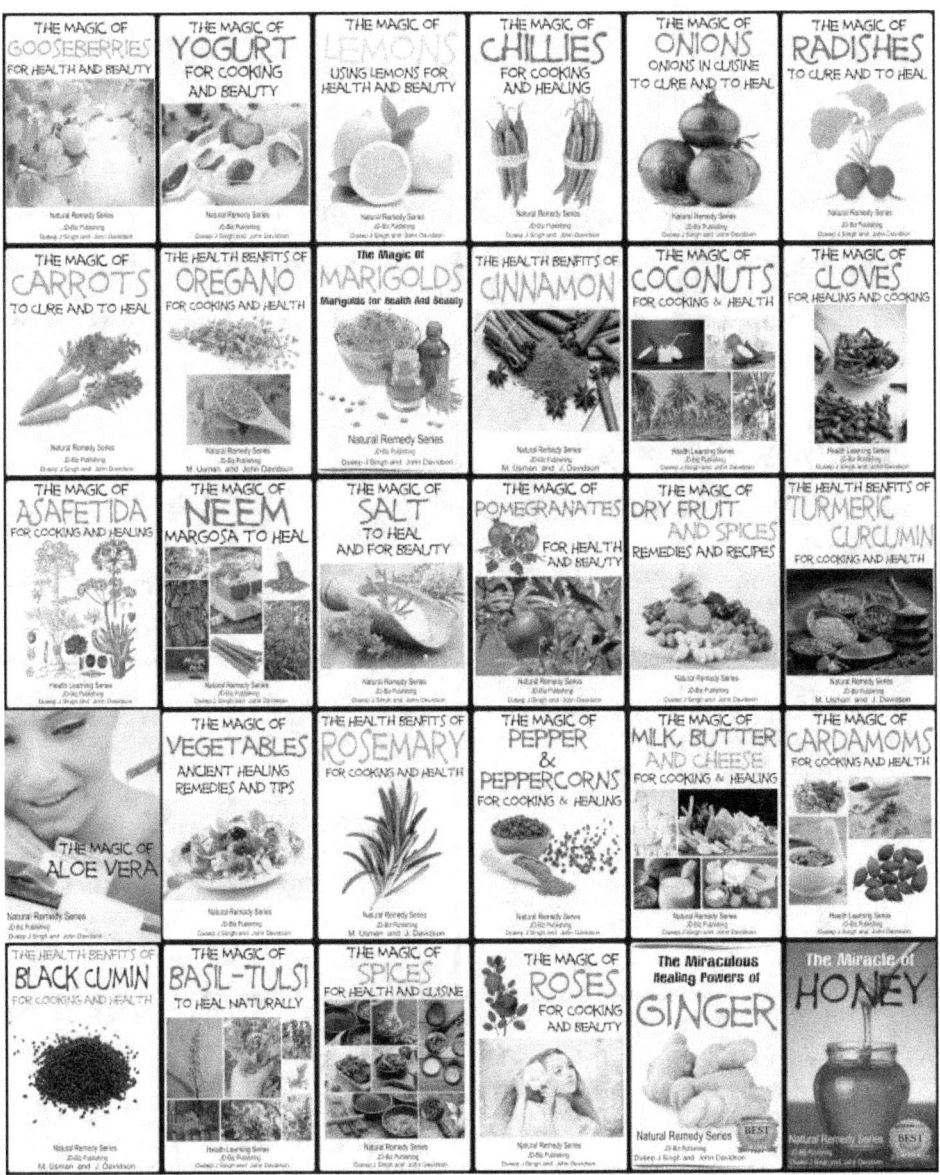

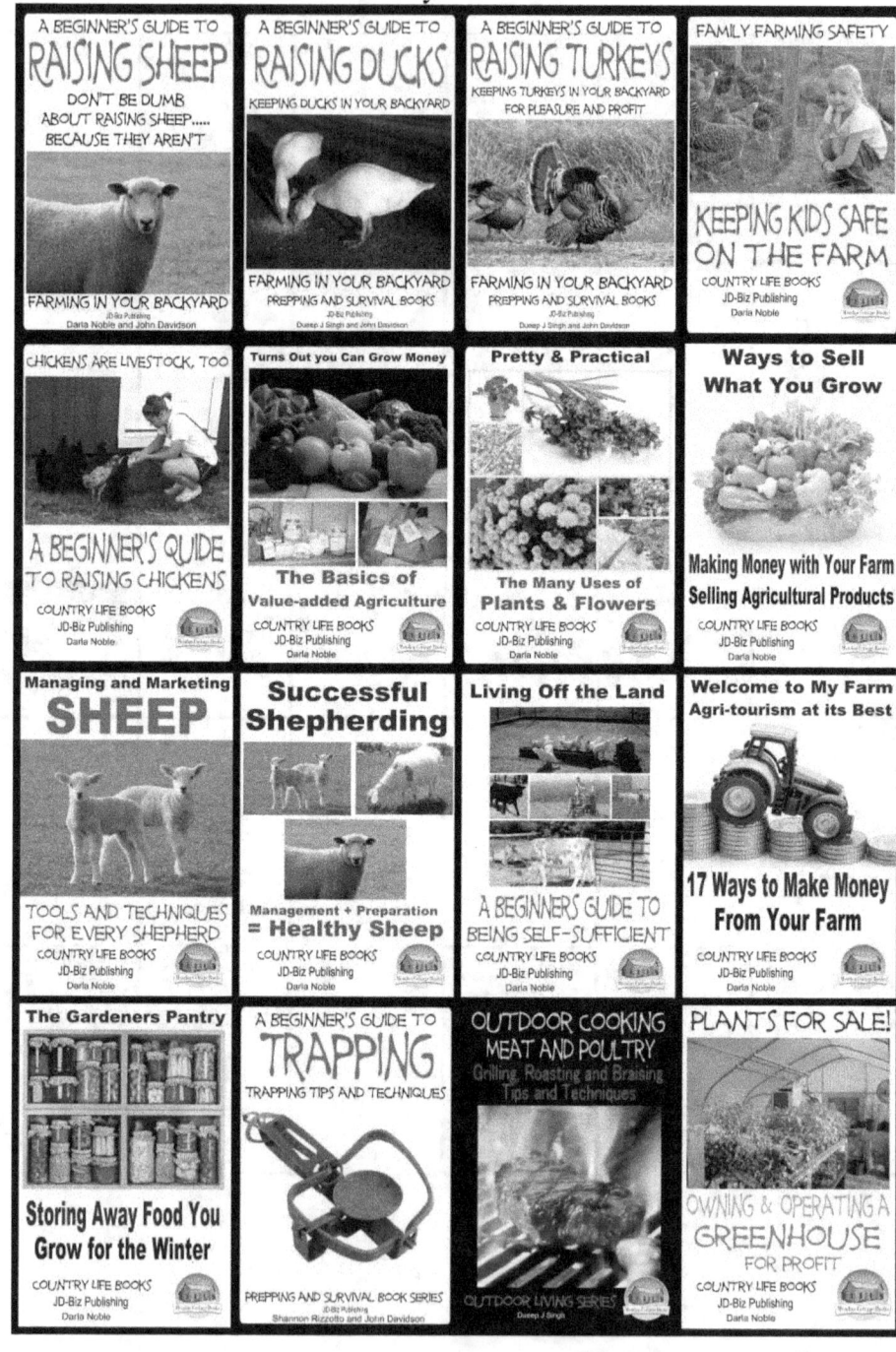

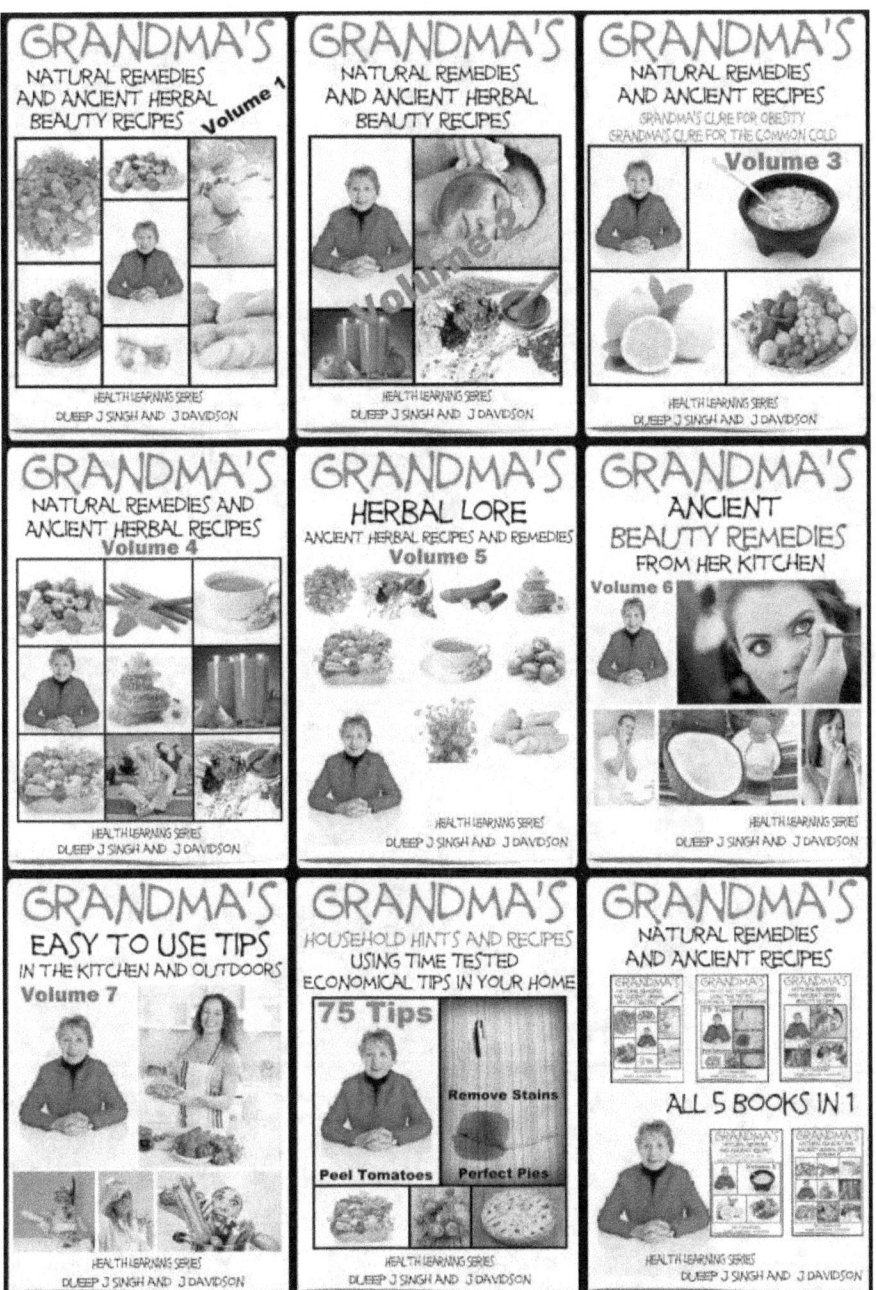

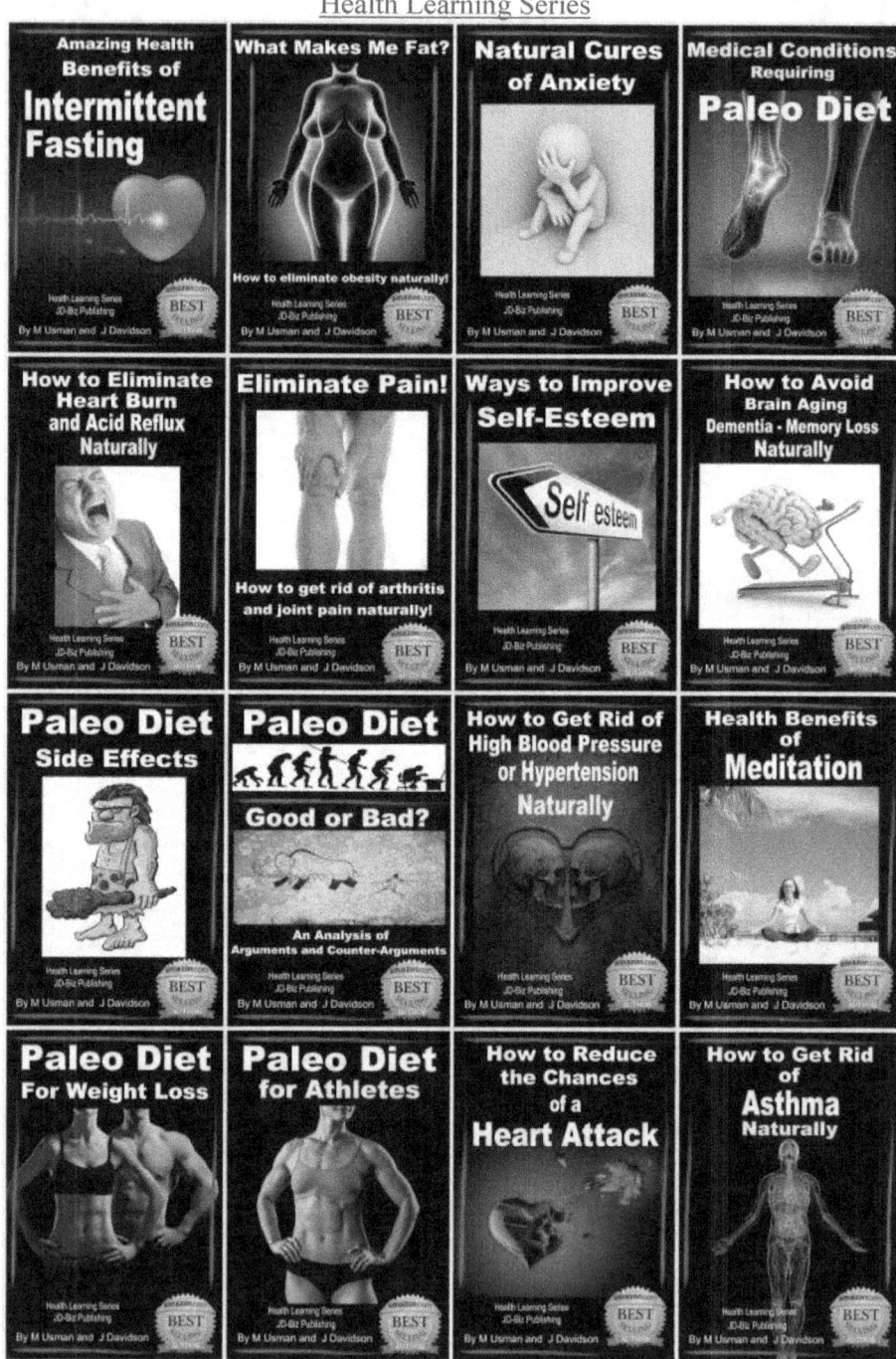

Amazing Animal Book Series

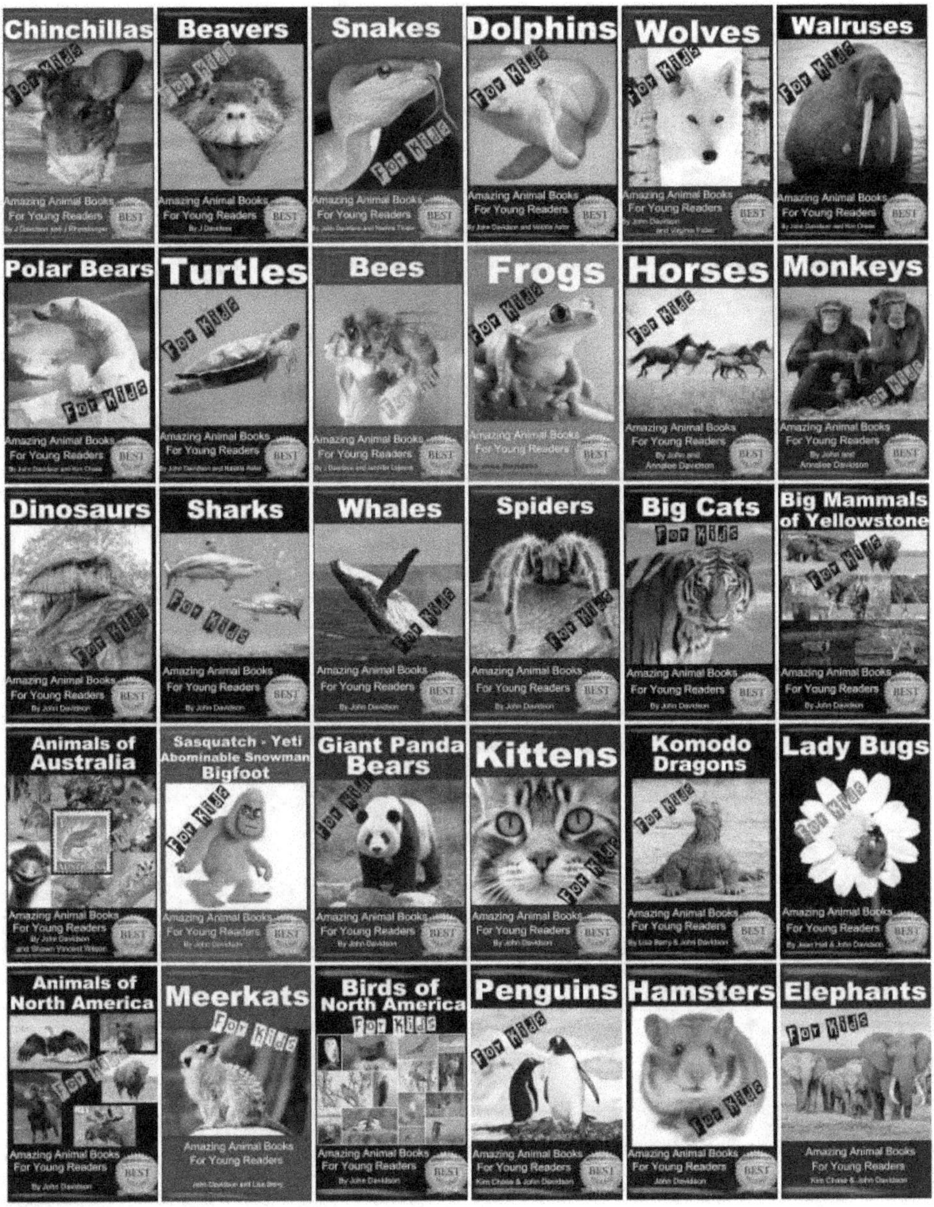

Learn To Draw Series

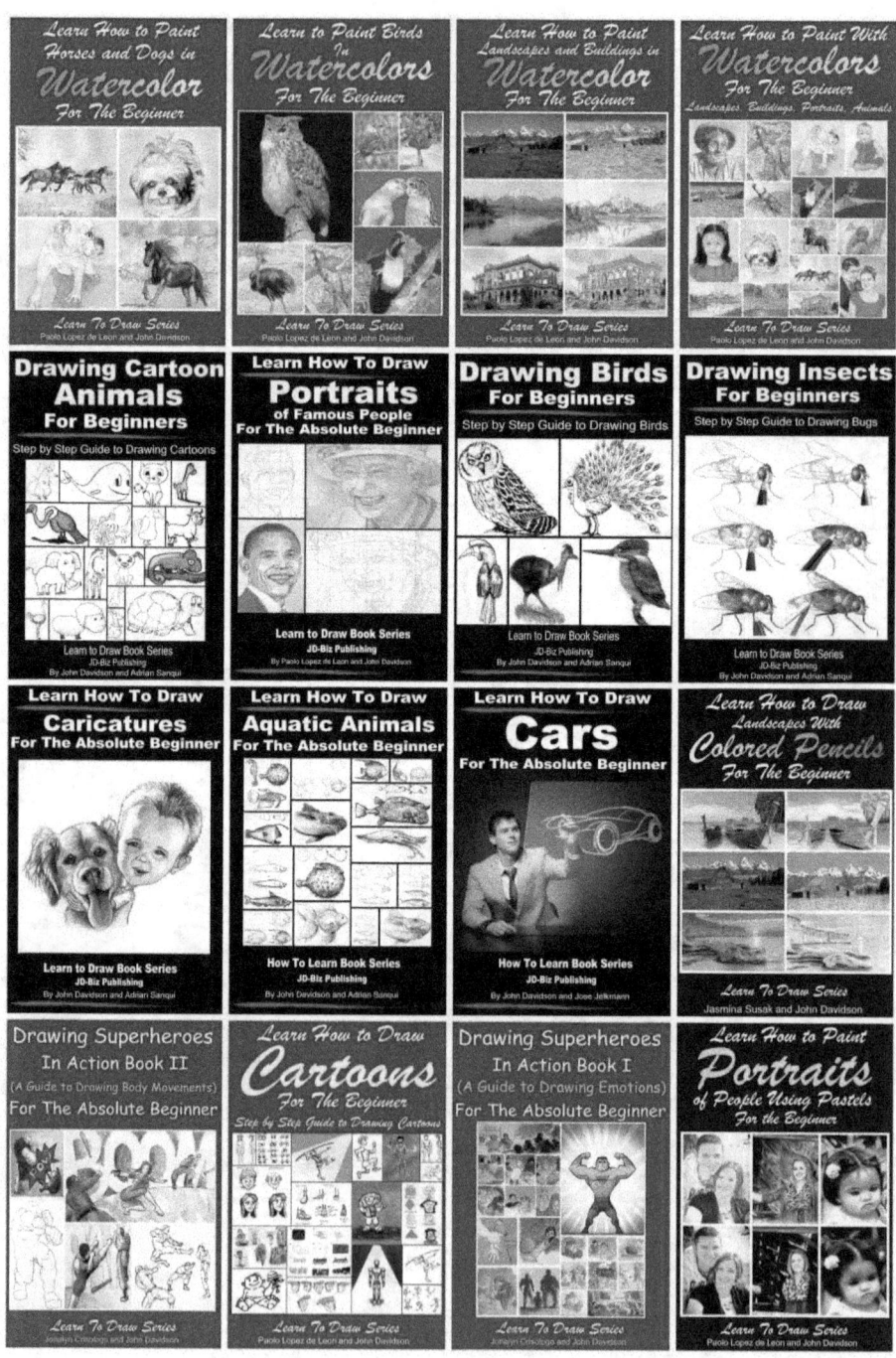

How to Build and Plan Books

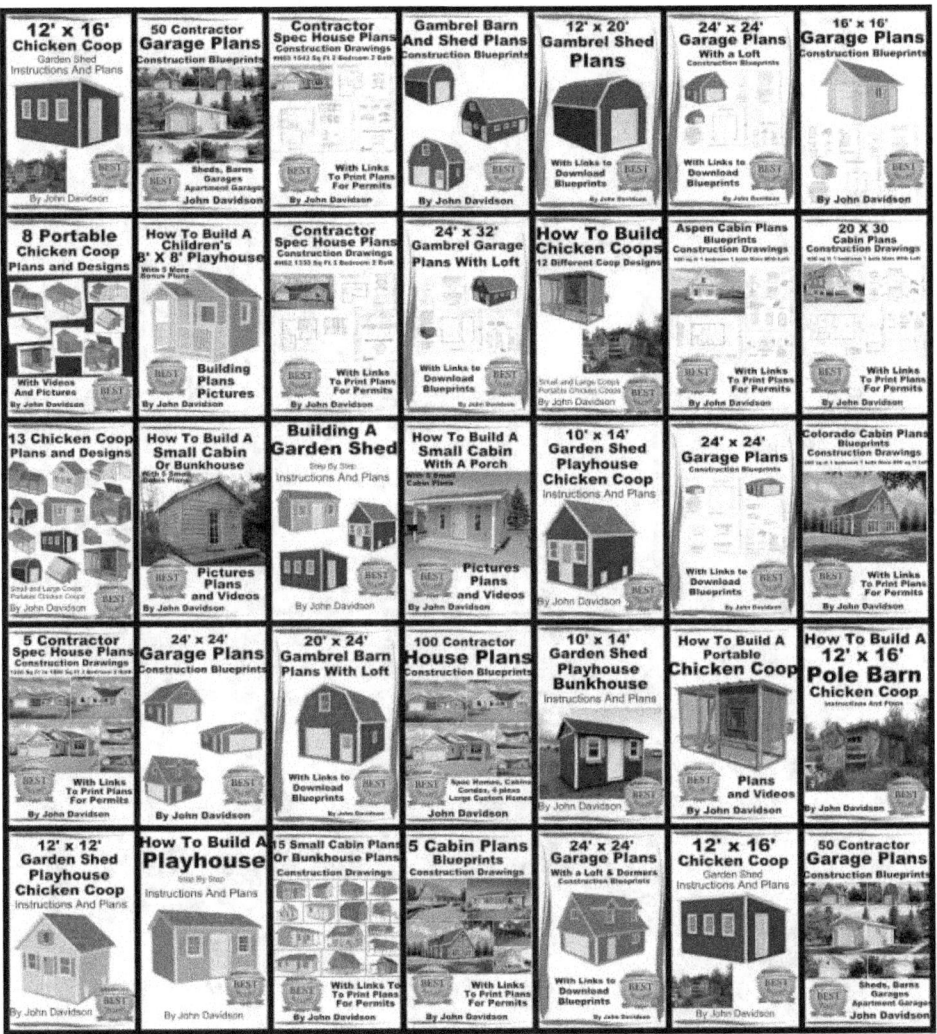

Entrepreneur Book Series

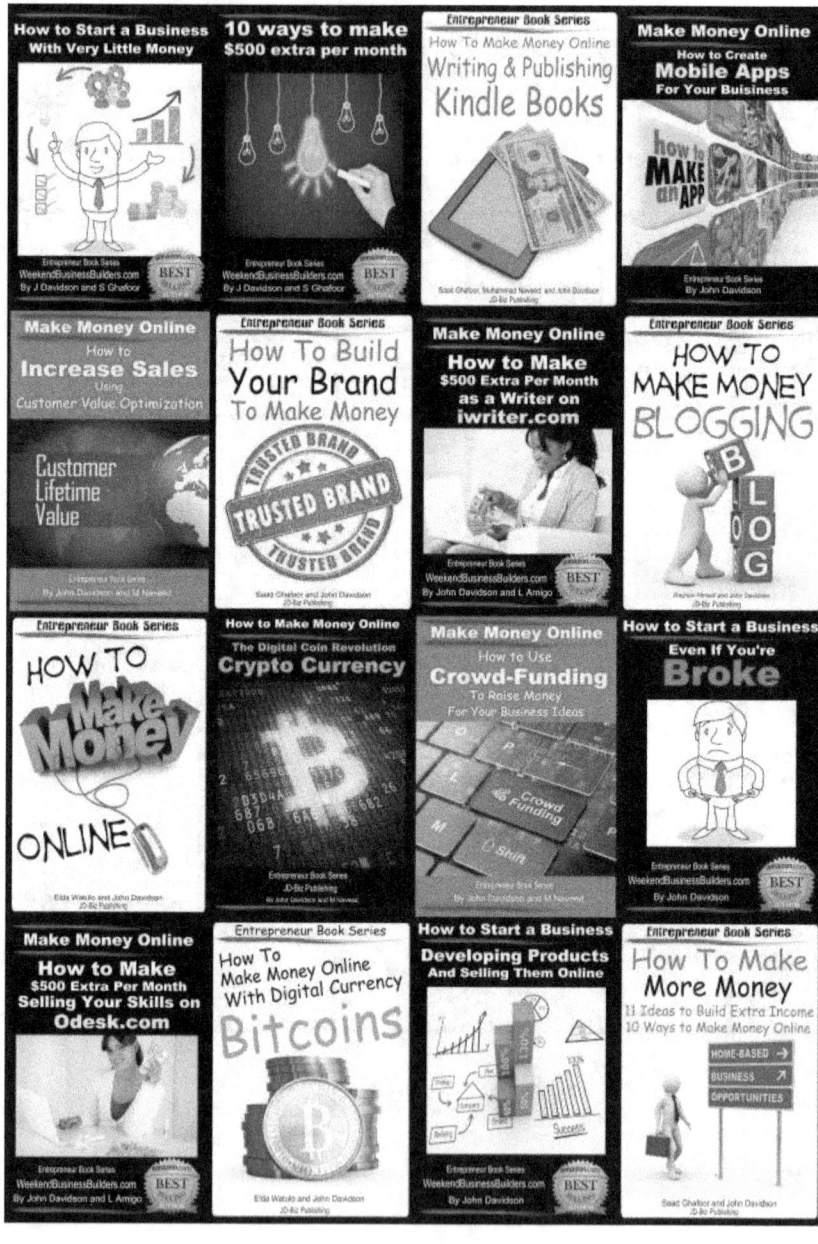

Our books are available at

1. Amazon.com

2. Barnes and Noble

3. Itunes

4. Kobo

5. Smashwords

6. Google Play Books

Publisher

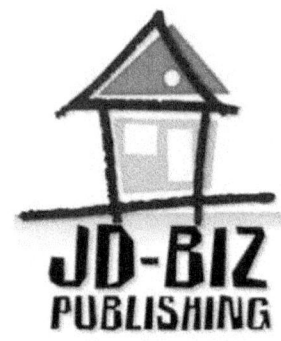

JD-Biz Corp

P O Box 374

Mendon, Utah 84325

http://www.jd-biz.com/

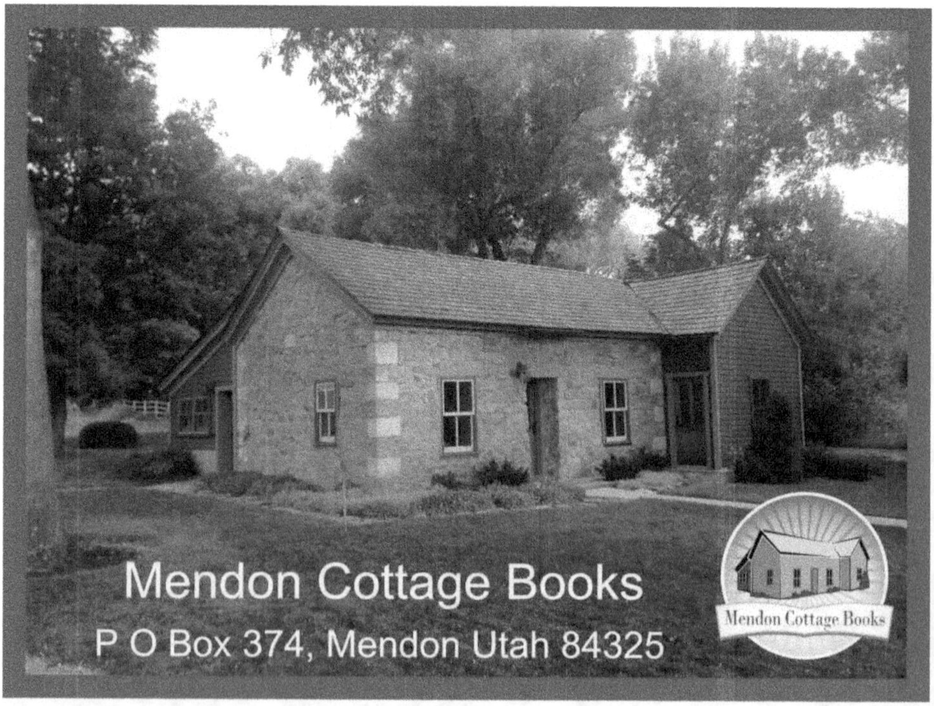

Mendon Cottage Books

P O Box 374, Mendon Utah 84325

Mendon Cottage Books

www.ingramcontent.com/pod-product-compliance
Lightning Source LLC
Chambersburg PA
CBHW070335290526
45791CB00003B/1337